I0419847

Organic Herbal Remedies to Help Treat Today's Common Ailments

Enjoy the Amazing Benefits of Natural Herbal Cures

By Byron Shu

Introduction

I want to thank you and congratulate you for downloading the book, "Organic Herbal Remedies to Help Treat Today's Common Ailments—Enjoy the Amazing Benefits of Natural Herbal Cures".

This book contains proven steps and strategies on how to remedy some of the most common diseases with organic foods and herbs.

It may sound cliché but it is true that prevention is unquestionably better than the most expensive and sophisticated treatment there is. Diseases such as hypertension, cancer and stroke affect the world today, but these can also be prevented. Though genetics may play a role in the development of these disorders, a large part of them is still linked to environmental factors such as diet, activity, smoking, alcoholism, and exposure to certain chemicals. What is surprising is that some of these diseases do not need the most advanced medicine or therapy to be cured. Sometimes, all they need is a healthy lifestyle.

One of the ways by which man can achieve a healthy body and prevent and treat ailments is by eating good foods. This eBook provides you with information about these foods and how they can protect your mind and body from diseases.

Thanks again for downloading this book, I hope you enjoy it!

Why You Should Read This Book

This book will help you understand the importance of eating organic foods and guide you on how you can get rid of your ailments.

Copyright

Disclaimer

Table of Contents

Why I wrote this Book

Why You Should Read This Book

Introduction

Chapter 1 Organic Remedies for the Heart

Chapter 2 Organic Remedies for the Brain

Chapter 3 Organic Remedies for Cancer

Chapter 4 Organic Remedies for the Skin

Bonus Chapter Tips on How You Can Totally Get Rid of Your Ailment

Conclusion

Chapter 1

Organic Remedies for the Heart

The heart is one of the most vulnerable organs. Any changes in the components of the blood, in the caliber and integrity of the blood vessels, and in the rate of metabolism can greatly alter the function of the heart. Heart disease, despite aggressive treatments and in depth researches and clinical trials, remains to be the leading cause of death in the world. Not only does it cause physical ailments, but it also affects the productivity and quality of life of a person. A person who has chronic heart failure won't be able to live the way a healthy human being can. It is for this very reason that keeping one's heart healthy has become a top priority.

Despite the expensive medications and sophisticated methods of treatment, there are still a lot of people who are living with heart disease. It can be as simple as mild hypertension or as bad as coronary artery disease. One factor contributing to this phenomenon is lifestyle, which encompasses the type of diet that you have and the type of physical activities that you do.

The type of food that people eat can greatly influence their health; hence, it is but essential to choose them wisely. With the presence of several fast food chains, patisseries, clubs and bars, living a healthy life and eating a healthy diet seemed to have become a challenge. It is more common now to see people flocking over fast food counters than over organic food shops. Though these unhealthy foods may bring you temporary joy and satisfaction, they do not, however, bring you good health. It is very important that people realize the beneficial effects of organic foods and herbs to their health.

Here are some of the best organic foods and herbs that can keep your heart robustly pumping:

1. Beans

Fill your heart with gladness with all the vitamins and minerals that beans can offer. They are not just rich in vitamin B complex and magnesium, but they are definitely rich in fiber as well. Fiber is a non-soluble product of certain vegetables and fruits that help facilitate digestion. But aside from protecting your stomach and your intestines from constipation, fiber also helps protect your heart from high levels of cholesterol and high blood pressure. Studies have shown that there is an inverse relationship between intake of beans and risk of heart diseases, particularly myocardial infarction (MI), which is also known as heart attack.

A daily serving of beans, whether white, black, or red, is associated with 30-40% reduction in the risk of MI. Researchers found out that there are various mechanisms by which beans help the heart but the most popular theory is the legumes' action on cholesterol. It is said that fiber binds cholesterol, in the form of bile, in the intestines and promotes it excretion. This bile, which is mainly composed of cholesterol, is deposited out of the body instead of being reabsorbed. This then leads to decreased cholesterol levels in the blood and decreased risk of heart attack!

2. Oatmeal

This famous hearty breakfast staple is well-loved not just because it is easy to prepare, but because it is truly healthy! Aside from being a flexible breakfast meal, since you can pair it with almost anything, eating oatmeal for breakfast has another advantage. Packed with omega-3 fatty acids, there is nothing more that you could ask for in a breakfast meal. Oats are cereal grains that are infused with nutrients and fiber.

There are two ways by which oats protect you from cardiovascular diseases. First is through beta-glucan, a type of fiber that is present in oats; and second is through the presence of antioxidants called avenenthramides that are considered to be unique to them. Beta-glucan, just like the type of fiber found in beans, helps lower blood cholesterol levels. It was found out that a bowl of oatmeal a day translates to a decrease in total cholesterol levels by almost 20% or a 40% reduction in the risk of developing heart diseases. Beta-glucan is also associated with lower levels of blood glucose, hence, help prevent Diabetes Mellitus.

Avenenthramides, on the other hand, are antioxidants that also help in lowering blood cholesterol levels by preventing the oxidation of LDL levels. LDL or low density lipoprotein is a type of cholesterol that transports fats from the liver to the cells. It is associated with several cardiovascular ailments, hence is called the bad cholesterol.

Avenenthramides also have anti-inflammatory properties which can help protect your blood vessels.

3. Walnuts

Aside from adding texture and taste to your cakes and other dishes, walnuts also do a good job of lowering your blood cholesterol levels. However, its blood cholesterol-lowering properties are not just limited to its high fiber content. Walnuts can lower blood cholesterol levels in several other ways.

First, it can increase the levels of the good cholesterol, a lipid-lowering mechanism that is entirely different from that of oatmeal. High density lipoprotein or HDL is the body's good cholesterol. It transports fats from the cells to the liver for metabolism. To put it simply, HDL binds cholesterol molecules that are present in the blood vessels and then brings them to the liver for breakdown. Cholesterol can cause an obstruction and blockade of the flow of blood if not removed.

Second, it improves the functioning of your blood vessels. As you have already learned, a change in the integrity and structure of blood vessels can significantly alter heart functioning.

Third, it contains ALA and Vitamin E that can effectively lower lipid levels. Alpha-linoleic acid is a type of polyunsaturated fatty acid that can be easily degraded by the enzymes in the gastrointestinal tract. This property of unsaturated fatty acids prevents them from solidifying under normal body temperature. Hence, these fatty acids are unlikely to deposit in the blood pipes and cause an obstruction.

4. Kale

Kale belongs to the family of cruciferous vegetables. It may only contain a few calories, approximately 40 Kcal, but it is definitely rich in vitamins and minerals. Kale contains high levels of magnesium, iron and potassium, which are all good for the heart. The major vitamins that you can get from kale are vitamins A, C and K, which are all important in the prevention of not only cardiovascular diseases, but also diseases of the brain and the kidneys. It is also high in fiber, which makes it a good cholesterol-lowering agent.

Vitamin C is popular for being an immune booster, but did you know that it also helps in maintaining the structure of your blood vessels? Vitamin C is a precursor in the synthesis of collagen, which is an important component of your blood vessels. Without collagen, blood vessels easily lose their elasticity, which is a risk factor for hypertension and aneurysms. Kale also comes with a lot of antioxidants that can prevent vascular damage.

5. Garlic

Probably one of the most famous super foods for the heart is garlic. The use of garlic as an antihypertensive agent has been recognized worldwide. More and more researches are still being conducted to discover more of its beneficial properties. In contrast to the other organic yields mentioned above, garlic does not contain high amounts of fiber to significantly lower blood cholesterol levels. Instead, it comes with heaping amounts of antioxidants and other compounds that do the trick.

What are these compounds? First, garlic contains polysulphides that prevent the constriction of blood vessels and inhibit the action of angiotensin II, a protein which is notorious for elevating the blood pressure. These polysuphides are converted to hydrogen sulphides that are mainly responsible for garlic's blood pressure-lowering effect. These sulphides increase the diameter of the blood vessels, a process called vasodilation, to allow more blood to flow through the tube. Garlic also has antioxidants that prevent damage to the blood vessels and natural anticoagulants that prevent formation of clots. These clots, when formed, can obstruct the passageway of blood, such as in the coronary arteries, leading to heart attack.

Chapter 2

Organic Remedies for the Brain

It is true that as people get older, various functions of the body gradually decline. The muscles get weaker, the vision gets blurred, the ears get less sensitive to sound, and the blood vessels get less elastic over time, thus leading to various diseases that predispose the elderly to injuries. The same is true for the brain. Neurons die and the connections between these cells degenerate leading to gradual decline in cognition. With aging, there is impairment of short- and long-term memory, sensory and motor functions.

Though aging cannot be stopped from happening, its onset and progression can, however, be delayed. Well, aside from the anti-aging supplements and memory enhancers that you can buy from the market, there are still a lot of things that you can do to protect your brain from degenerative diseases, such as Alzheimer's and Parkinson's disease. Several studies have established the role of organic herbs and foods in keeping the brain healthy.

Here are some of the herbs that can enhance the functions of your hardworking brain:

1. **Broccoli**

   Boost your brain power by eating a serving of broccoli every day. Just like Kale, broccoli belongs to the family of cruciferous vegetables which are known for their enormous antioxidant, vitamin, and mineral content. Broccoli contains a lot of compounds that have been shown to help delay the progression of degeneration of brain cells. One of them is lignan, which is a phytonutrient that has been known to act specifically on the brain. It boosts cognitive functions by improving one's learning capabilities, memory, and reasoning.

   It is also rich in glucosinate, which is a compound that prevents the decrease in the levels of acetylcholine, a chemical mediator in several brain processes, such as movement and memory. A decrease in the levels of this neurotransmitter has been implicated in the development of Alzheimer's disease.

2. **Avocado**

   Avocado had been in the dark for quite some time because of several misconceptions. It was initially believed to be unhealthy because of its high fat content. However, it was later on revealed that though they may be fatty, the types of fat it contains are not harmful at all. They were actually high density lipoproteins and omega- 3 fatty acids. Because of this, avocado has become the subject of researches that aim to study its beneficial effects.

Currently, avocado is known to contain a lot of nutrients, not only the fats mentioned above. It is rich in vitamin B complex (B1, B2, B3, B5, B6, B9, and B12), which is known to be neuroprotective, vitamin E, which is a potent scavenger for free radicals, and vitamins A, D, K and C, which all have beneficial effects not only to the brain but to other organs as well.

How does avocado protect the brain? First, the fat content of this fruit allows for good blood circulation in the brain. Omega-3 fatty acid has an anti-inflammatory property that protects the blood vessels from damage. Because HDLs facilitate the removal of cholesterol plaques from the lumen of the blood vessels, adequate blood flow to the various regions of the brain is achieved. This prevents stroke from occurring. Stroke is a consequence of decreased delivery of oxygen to the brain, which happens when there is occlusion of blood vessels.

Second, omega-3 fatty acids are associated with better mood. Studies found out that there is actually an inverse relationship between the levels of omega-3 fatty acids in the blood and the risk of depression and hostility. There is, on the other hand, a direct relationship between one's intelligence quotient (IQ) and omega-3 fatty acid levels.

And third, the vitamin K content of avocado protects the brain from hemorrhage. Vitamin K is needed in the activation of several clotting factors and deficiency of this vitamin can lead to excessive bleeding.

3. Coconut oil

Just like avocado, coconut oil has received a bad welcome from many health experts for the past few years because of its fat content. However, these speculations have been proven to be wrong. Coconut oil is trans-fat free. Trans-fat is a type of saturated fat that is known to cause several heart ailments. Unlike unsaturated fats, saturated fats solidify or precipitate under normal body temperature. Hence, they have a great tendency to form aggregates inside the blood vessels and cause obstruction.

Sticking to the walls of the vessel does not only cause obstruction of the flow of blood but it also stimulates the inflammatory process. In an attempt of the body to get rid of these sticky fats, the inflammatory cells and the platelets surround the plaque causing further harm. The more cells come into the site of obstruction, the more obstructed the vessel will become. Occlusion leads to decreased blood flow to the brain, which in turn leads to death of brain cells. With the death of these cells, the brain is less able to perform its functions.

Supplementation with coconut oil has also been found out to be very beneficial for people suffering from Alzheimer's type of dementia. Researchers claim that coconut oil can actually protect the brain cells from the damaging effects of a protein called beta-amyloid. These proteins are seen in patients with Alzheimer's disease as cellular deposits and have been implicated in the production of cognitive deficits typical of the said disease.

4. Spinach

As a child, you might have already appreciated the importance and health benefits of this herb as you watched Popeye the Sailorman's muscles get pumped up after dumping a canfull of spinach into his mouth. However, you might not have realized then that there is still a lot more to spinach than being a muscle-pumper.

Spinach is loaded with several micronutrients making it an all-in-one green leafy vegetable. It is packed with antioxidants making it a good anti-aging agent. It is also infused with multiple vitamins and minerals that make it an energy booster. Fiber is also etched in every corner of this vegetable. But the most important component of spinach that makes it a perfect brain food is folate or Vitamin B9.

Folic acid has long been used as a supplement by pregnant mothers as this can prevent the formation of spinal cord and brain abnormalities, called neural tube defects, in fetuses. These spinal and brain defects are commonly seen as masses of meninges and spinal cord herniating out of the skin of the back, usually in the lower portions. But the beneficial effects of folate are not only limited to fetuses and pregnant mothers, because everyone can benefit from its neuroprotective effects.

Folate promotes neural development, growth of new cells and formation of new connections among neurons. These connections are necessary for faster transmission of impulses to and from the brain. An increase in the level of this B vitamin is also associated with higher levels of neurotransmitters, most especially of dopamine and serotonin.

Dopamine is mainly responsible for motor functions, while serotonin is mainly responsible for the regulation of one's mood and sleep pattern. Serotonin is also the neurotransmitter that is implicated in sundown phenomenon, a disorder that is characterized by depressed mood during sunset and a manic or normal mood in the presence of sunlight. It was theorized that sunlight induces the production of serotonin leading to enhanced mood. Aside from spinach, folate can also be found in eggplant, celery and beans.

5. Olive Oil

Olive oil is not just great for cooking pastas, but it is also great in protecting your brain from age-related degeneration. Olive oil, just like avocado and coconut oil, is rich in polyunsaturated fats. Aside from preventing stroke, polyunsaturated fats promote the transmission of impulses to and from the nervous system. Fats facilitate myelination of nerves.

Normally, the brain transmits several signals within a second because of the presence of myelin sheath. This sheath does not only serve as protective covering of your nerves, but they also facilitate faster transmission of impulses. Without them, transmission will be disrupted and slower. An impulse normally travels through nerve A, then nerve B, then nerve C before it reaches its destination. However, if a person has deficient myelin, an impulse will not traverse its normal route. It can either go to nerve Z or to nerve A before it can reach its target cell. Olive oil also has a role in the regulation of one's mood.

Chapter 3

Organic Remedies for Cancer

Despite recent advancements in chemotherapy, radiotherapy and targeted therapy, cancer still has remained to be one of the greatest threats to man. It is one of the 5 leading causes of morbidity and mortality worldwide. Cancer is one of the most feared diseases of man and it still continues to hunt people down. Unlike other diseases, cancer does not have certain predilections. It equally happens among men and women, young and old, and rich and poor.

Though there have already been theories regarding its development, a lot is still not known about its cause. Yes, it is true that carcinogens are one of the main culprits behind this debilitating disease, but the main mechanism behind its origin still remains to be discovered.

Cancer is characterized by unrelenting proliferation and growth of abnormal cells that tend to invade other organs in a process called metastasis. Though much of the efforts of researches have been geared towards its cure or control, the importance of prevention cannot be emphasized enough. Cancer makes you realize that an ounce of prevention is really better than a pound of cure.

One of the preventive measures that are being advised nowadays is the adaptation of a healthy lifestyle, which encompasses healthy diet, regular exercise, and avoidance of smoking and alcohol. One of the first few cancers that have been associated with poor diet is colon cancer. It was found out that people who eat more fats, more meat, more processed foods and less vegetables and fruits are more prone to developing colorectal malignancy than those who do not. Since then, having a well-balanced diet has been advocated diligently.

What are some of the organic remedies for cancer?

1. Berries

The family of berries, which includes blueberries, strawberries, raspberries and cranberries, can be considered to be the most popular anti-cancer organic agent. They have long been known to contain phytochemicals such as anthocyanins, flavonoids, catechins and resveratrol, which are all potent antioxidants. These phytochemicals were found to be associated with lower rates of inflammation not only in the gastrointestinal tract but in other organs as well. How does inflammation cause cancer?

An organ that is regularly exposed to inflammation will try to find a way to protect itself from the damaging effects of the inflammatory cells. One of its protective measures is to undergo metaplasia, a condition that is characterized by transformation of a normal cell into a different type of cell.

For example, the esophagus is normally lined with a type of epithelium called stratified squamous, a multiple layer of flat cells. However, with chronic irritation, such as with frequent reflux of acid from the stomach to the esophagus, this squamous epithelium can transform into columnar cells, a type of epithelium that has greater resilience against the destructive effects of gastric acid. This can lead to more transformations down the line, until they ultimately transform into tumor cells. Reducing the incidence of inflammation can protect the esophagus and the other organs against metaplasia and eventually, cancer.

Berries were also found to be linked with reduction in the levels of free radicals, which are metabolic byproducts that induce damage to the cellular DNA. One's damage to DNA occurs, uninhibited growth and proliferation take place, circumventing and overcoming the natural growth regulators of the body. Berries help by inducing death of these cancer cells and regulation of their growth.

2. Grapefruit

Grapefruit, just like blueberries, is also loaded with antioxidants, one of which is vitamin C or ascorbic acid. This vitamin has been known to be an immune booster, which means that it helps ward off infections and promote wound healing. But you might be wondering how vitamin C can prevent cancer or inhibit its growth. Vitamin C can inhibit the formation of nitrogen compounds that are said to be carcinogenic.

Another potent antioxidant that grapefruit contains is naringenin, and is probably the major source of its anti-cancer property. Aside from scavenging free radicals, it also has anti-inflammatory properties, as well as the ability to regulate metabolism of carbohydrates and function of the immune system.

One of the main mechanisms by which mutation occurs is oxidative damage to the cellular DNA and studies have found out that daily intake of grapefruit leads to reduction in the amount of oxidative damage by more than 20 percent. One unique feature of naringenin is its ability to reduce the release of hepatitis C virus from the liver cells. This virus, along with Hepatitis B virus, is a risk factor for the development of hepatocellular carcinoma. Though more studies are needed to prove it, this finding is considered promising.

3. Turmeric

Another well-loved organic remedy is turmeric, which belongs to the family of ginger. This crop is not only used in preventing cancer, but it is also widely used in several ailments ranging from simple cough and colds to more complex diseases, such as diabetes mellitus. This could be attributed to its active component, curcumin.

This compound has been known to have potent anti-inflammatory and antioxidant properties. Curcumin inhibits cancer in two ways: first, it specifically targets cancer cells without causing harm to the healthy ones. And second, curcumin can augment the anti-cancer effects of certain chemotherapeutic drugs.

Cancer cells are known for their invasiveness and metastatic property. Due to their uncontrolled growth, cancer cells tend to steal the nutrients that are supposed to be delivered to the normal cells. However, these nutrients become less adequate for the growing tumor; hence the cancer cells will find a way to increase its nutrient supply.

The first thing that cancer cells will do is to promote the formation of new blood vessels, a process called angiogenesis, through the release of certain growth factors, such as PDGF and VEGF. The formation of these new blood vessels translates to more blood and nutrient supply. If these mechanisms were not enough, the cells will then try to look for other places where it could get adequate amounts of nutrients. This is where metastasis comes in.

Through the newly-formed blood vessels, the cancer cells are able to travel to different sites and establish another mass. What curcumin does is that it prevents angiogenesis from occurring, inhibiting these cells from migrating to distant locations and the tumor from profusely growing. As a result, the tumor cells die and the tumor shrinks in size.

4. Spinach

You have already learned how spinach protects the brain from degeneration. Spinach also inhibits the progression of cancer. Spinach has been specifically studied for the treatment of breast and ovarian cancers. Studies have shown that spinach contains antioxidants and phytochemicals that are effective in impeding the proliferation and growth of breast cancer cells.

Spinach is also rich in glycolipids which have been shown to have inhibitory effects on the DNA enzyme involved in cell division. This enzyme, called the DNA polymerase enzyme, catalyzes replication of genes. Hence, if uncontrolled, mutated genes will continue to replicate and cause further harm to the body. Daily intake of spinach has been shown to reduce incidence of colorectal malignancy by as much as 50 percent.

5. Green Tea

Nothing could be more relaxing than drinking a cup of green tea while reading your favorite book or while chatting with your friends. Many people say that green has some calming effects, making it a favorite drink during breakfast or break times. But this effect of green tea only makes up a small percentage of its healing potential. The benefits of green tea are not just limited to relaxation and to the skin; rather, they are also linked with reduction in the incidence of various diseases such as cancer, especially of the stomach, rectum and pancreas.

The quest for green tea's health benefits started when it had been observed that among people who regularly drink tea, there are only a small percentage that develops cancer versus the large percentage among people who do not. The component of green tea that is implicated in cancer prevention is catechin, a form of polyphenol that has antioxidant property. Catechins are said to kill tumor cells by inducing cellular damage and inhibit new blood vessels from forming. Other types of teas, such as black and oolong are said to have the same effects as that of green.

Chapter 4

Organic Remedies for the Skin

The skin is the body's primary defense mechanism against invading and infective microorganisms. Though it may have its own ways of defending itself against these stubborn agents, the skin deserves some special attention as well.

There are a lot of ways by which your skin can get damaged. First, there is the sun that emits UV rays causing damage to your cells. The UV rays and frequent sun exposure are implicated in the development of several skin carcinomas, such as melanoma, squamous cell carcinoma and basal cell carcinoma.

Second, the skin, due to its location, is prone to blunt and sharp injuries. Skin can be easily punctured, cut, lacerated and inflamed. These cause break in the continuity of skin predisposing it to various infections.

And third, the skin can also get damaged with decreased blood supply. This is most especially true for people who are living in cold mountains or in freezing temperatures. Under cold temperature, the body tends to direct the flow of blood towards the more vital organs, such as the heart and the brain while leaving only a small amount of blood to circulate in the peripheries. The initial sign of this compensatory response is pallor. However, this could get worse and lead to total absence of blood supply causing necrosis or death of skin cells.

Other skin conditions that might get you worried are acne, eczema, and infections. The good news is that there are several organic herbs and foods that you can eat or apply to protect your skin from these harmful environmental factors.

1. Tomato

One of the most popular ingredients in several skin care products is tomato. This red fruit is popular for its lycopene which is another type of antioxidant. Lycopene does not only give tomato its rich red color, but it also provides tomato its healing and anti-aging properties. You have already learned that free radicals are byproducts of oxidation-reduction reactions that can damage cellular DNA, a mechanism of cancer development. But aside from damaging your DNA, these free radicals also accelerate the aging process by causing oxidative stress.

Tomato helps fight skin aging by neutralizing these stubborn free radicals. Tomato is rich in Vitamin A which does not only improve one's eyesight but can also make the skin glow. Vitamin A also stimulates the formation of collagen, which is an important precursor to a youthful skin. Not only that!

Tomatoes can also protect the skin from the damaging effects of the UV rays by providing sun protection factor of 1.3.

2. Oatmeal

The beneficial effects of oatmeal are truly limitless for it can also be used in several skin ailments. Oats are usually applied onto the skin for its hydrating and exfoliating effects. Oats also absorb excess oil from your skin without dehydrating it. If you are suffering from skin irritation or simple itchiness, then you can go for a short oatmeal bath.

Skin irritations are usually caused by excessive oiliness or excessive dryness. When irritated, the skin tends to be itchy and more inflamed. Itchiness then prompts you to scratch that small portion of your skin until it is relieved. However, the danger here is that you can get a layer of your skin abraded. Oats help you relieve itchiness and irritation by mildly moisturizing your skin. They also contain saponin which is great for its cleansing properties.

3. Orange

Have you ever wondered why some people put orange peels on their faces? This is because orange peels are rich in vitamins and minerals. You would even be surprised to know that peels contain higher levels of ascorbic acid than the fruit itself!

Orange has a wide range of beneficial effects to the skin. Aside from giving your skin a youthful glow, oranges are also used in treating acne, reducing wrinkle lines, and eliminating those stubborn blackheads. Orange peels help prevent acne from forming by cleaning your pores and stripping off excess sebum or oil. The presence of too much oil makes your pore a good breeding ground for bacteria. This then causes inflammation, and eventually acne.

If your main concern is your fine wrinkle lines on your forehead or around your eyes, then oranges can definitely help you. Orange contains citric acid, a component of AHA, which is a potent exfoliator and anti-aging compound. This helps smoothen out wrinkles and brighten up your skin tone!

4. Kiwi

This fruit may be small but its beneficial effects are never-ending. This fruit is teeming with several vitamins that act as antioxidants. A single kiwi fruit contains the highest level of vitamin C, as well as vitamin E. Aside from neutralizing free radicals, vitamin C is also known for hastening wound healing. This is through its effects on the hydroxylation of a compound called proline which is involved in the repair of cells and tissues.

As mentioned in the previous chapters, ascorbic acid plays an essential role in the production of collagen, which is not only needed by the blood vessels but by the skin as well. Collagen is a major component of the matrix of the skin cells. This matrix provides stability to the skin structure, as well as nutrients. Collagen and elastin work together to keep the skin taut and as a result, the skin looks more naturally youthful.

5. Witch Hazel

Sounds familiar, doesn't it? This is because witch hazel extract is a popular ingredient in several skin care products. It has been used as an anti-inflammatory, antimicrobial and a moisturizing agent since time immemorial. Due to these properties of witch hazel, it has been used to relieve itchiness, rashes and infections, such as impetigo. One of the most remarkable benefits of witch hazel is its ability to hasten wound healing and improve vascular tone, which makes it effective for skin conditions like eczema. This has been shown to be attributed to one of its active components, called tannins. Witch hazel can also be used to soothe sunburns.

Bonus Chapter

Tips on How You Can Totally Get Rid of Your Ailments

Eating organic foods is one step toward living a healthy life but you should not stop here. There are other steps that you must take in order to achieve a healthy body, mind and spirit. Here are some tips on how you can live to the fullest and enjoy an illness-free life:

1. **Get some exercise.** This might sound a cliché and this might not sound so good to you, but there is really nothing better than the combination of a healthy diet and regular exercise. A healthy diet will give you all the nutrients that your body needs to function well while regular exercise will augment your metabolic processes and facilitate several mechanisms that can protect your organs from several disorders.

   Getting some exercise does not mean that you have to go to the gym every day. You can do some simple exercises such as walking for 20 to 30 minutes every day. You can accomplish this through several ways. You can walk your way to your workplace or you can park your car a little farther from the entrance of your office. Upon waking up or before going to bed, you can do simple stretching exercises just enough to make you sweat and release the tension on your muscles.

2. **Avoid or stop smoking and alcohol.** Give yourself a pat on the back if you don't smoke. But if you do, still give yourself a pat on the back and tell yourself, "I can stop this." Quitting smoking is definitely not an easy thing to do, especially if you have been smoking for quite some time now. But there is no reason for you to lose hope. There are a lot of people who have been through those difficult times and a lot of them have emerged victorious in their goal of totally quitting it. The same is true for drinking alcohol. How can you control yourself when you have friends calling you for a drink almost every night?

   There are three things that you will need to stop these unhealthy habits. You need time, motivation and help. You need time to prepare yourself for the quitting day; motivation that is firm enough to give you the strength to control your urges; and lastly, help from your family, friends and from your physician. You don't have to do this overnight. Quitting is a step-by-step process. It might take a while but the results would really be worth it. Here is one tip: Quitting smoking for 5 years restores your lungs to normal. It would be as if you have never even smoked in your life.

3. **Minimize intake of unhealthy foods.** Unhealthy foods come in different packages- there are instant noodles, canned goods, processed and cured meat, fatty dairy products, carbonated beverages, and a lot more. How do you know

whether they are healthy or not? The easiest way to check is by reading nutrition labels. If you have hypertension or any heart disease, it is advisable that you look for low-fat, zero sat-fat and zero trans-fat products, especially dairy products.

Looking at the sodium content of these foods also helps. The recommended daily intake of sodium is 2 grams or 2000 mg, which is approximately equal to one teaspoon of salt. Product labels would also show you the amount of specific vitamins and minerals that are present by giving you a percentage. For example, the label of a bottled orange juice reads vitamin C- 50%. This means that the amount of vitamin C that this bottle contains is 50% of your recommended daily allowance.

4. **De-stress.** Stress is one of the reasons why you have depressed immune function. Try to get some time to relax. When you are stressed, your body produces hormones, such as epinephrine, norepinephrine, and cortisol that promote the production of glucose or sugar and breakdown of fats. Though breakdown of fats seems a good effect, it actually leads to production of more free radicals. These hormones can also constrict your blood vessels which can lead to higher blood pressure. Practice yoga, travel, go out with your friends, or listen to music while reading a good book. These activities can help you de-stress.

Conclusion

The world may give you a lot of reasons to get sick, but there are surely a lot of ways for you to get healthy. These organic herbs do not just provide you with energy; rather, they nourish your body and protect it from diseases. There are still a lot more of them around. This time, it is not just apple that keeps the doctor away. Each vegetable, fruit, and herb is infused with vitamins, minerals, and a lot more healthy compounds that can keep you strong, happy, and healthy!

One Last Thing...

If you enjoyed this book or found it useful I'd be very grateful if you'd post a short review on Amazon. Your support really does make a difference and I read all the reviews personally so I can get your feedback and make this book even better.

If you'd like to leave a review then all you need to do is click the review link on this book's page...

Thank You so Much